ACNE

Acne Treatment
Acne Removal
Acne Remedies For Clear Skin

By Ace McCloud

Copyright © 2013

Disclaimer

The information provided in this book is designed to provide helpful information on the subjects discussed. This book is not meant to be used, nor should it be used, to diagnose or treat any medical condition. For diagnosis or treatment of any medical problem, consult your own physician. The publisher and author are not responsible for any specific health or allergy needs that may require medical supervision and are not liable for any damages or negative consequences from any treatment, action, application or preparation, to any person reading or following the information in this book. Any references included are provided for informational purposes only. Readers should be aware that any websites or links listed in this book may change.

Table of Contents

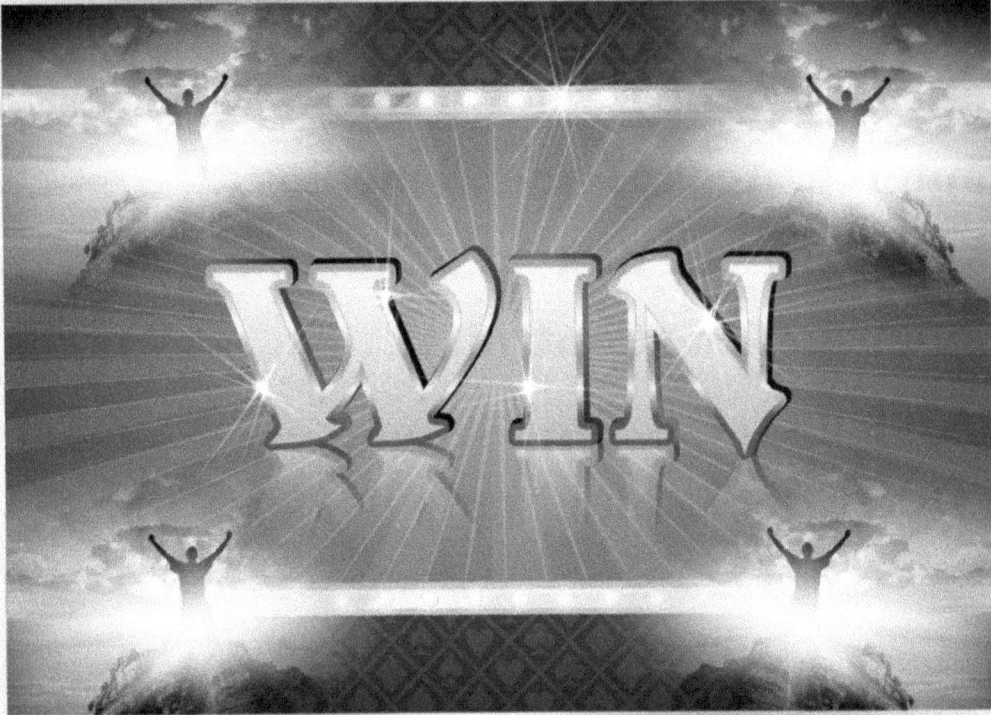

DEDICATED TO THOSE WHO ARE PLAYING THE GAME OF LIFE TO

WIN

KEEP ON PUSHING AND NEVER GIVE UP!

Ace McCloud

Be sure to check out my website for all my Books and Audio books.

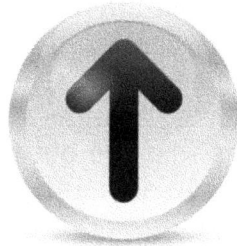

Introduction

I want to thank you and congratulate you for downloading this book. In the following pages you will discover proven steps and strategies that can help you easily reduce and eliminate acne.

Acne is a common skin condition that affects most people and it can persist late into life. Doing what doesn't work can leave you with unsightly scars and acne that will just not go away. Curing acne takes time, eating the right foods and the right use of products and treatments. You may be surprised at the number of all natural and inexpensive solutions that are out there for acne. In this book you will discover exactly what you need to do in order to end your acne problems once and for all!

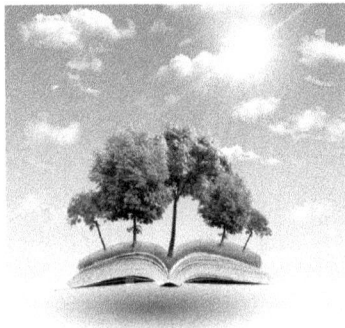

Chapter 1: Acne Treatment

Most people will only need treatment for mild acne. The common treatments for acne are over-the-counter medications. These products contain active ingredients that can kill acne causing bacteria and clean the pores to prevent acne.

Resorcinol

Resorcinol is a crystalline phenol that can dissolve whiteheads and blackheads. It improves the skin condition by breaking down the upper layer of skin where dirt is trapped. Unfortunately, resorcinol cannot kill bacteria nor does it prevent its buildup.

Benzoyl Peroxide

Benzoyl Peroxide is a common active ingredient in acne products. It can kill bacteria and reduce the oil production. Benzoyl is crystalline peroxide that is used in bleaching. It can also work as a peeling agent that accelerates the skin's shedding making the pores cleaner.

Salicylic Acid

Salicylic acid is effective in reducing inflammation. It causes skin to shed easily which makes room for new cells to grow. It prevents blackheads and whiteheads and reduces the production of oil.

Sulfur

Sulfur is a yellow crystalline solid in its natural form. It has been an ancient cure for acne, eczema and psoriasis. The elemental sulfur oxidizes to acid which can be an antibacterial agent.

Retin-A

Retin- A is an acne treatment which is derived from vitamin A. It is mostly used to treat mild to moderate acne. It is especially effective in eliminating whiteheads and blackheads. Retin-A works by speeding up the cell turnover and decrease the buildup of dead skin cells.

Azelaic Acid

Azelaic acid can be used for mild to moderate acne. It kills bacteria that can cause pimples and reduces the inflammation. Azelaic acid strengthens the cells and lines the follicles and stop oil eruptions. It is also recommended for people who suffer from melasma or dark spots that occur after the acne has healed.

Treating more severe cases of acne involves stronger medications that may need a prescription from a dermatologist. These prescription medicines can be in the form of creams, lotions, and pills.

Corticosteroid injection

If acne turns into a cyst and becomes severely inflamed, a dermatologist can inject a diluted form of corticosteroid to prevent the cyst from erupting and scarring. It also helps speed up the healing process.

Isotretinoin

Isotretinoin is prescribed for a severe cyst that antibiotics cannot handle. It is a powerful medication that is used when acne does not respond to common treatments. While it is very effective, it can also have severe side effects like birth defects for pregnant women, dry skin, and muscle aches. This drug should only be administered with the supervision of a specialist to avoid any dangerous effects.

Oral contraceptive

Oral contraceptives, like ethinyl estradiol, has been proven to decrease the acne of women. It can also cause side effects like breast tenderness and headaches. Women who want to use oral contraceptives as acne medication should consult their doctor first.

Antibiotics

Antibiotics are used for moderate to severe acne. However, people can build up a resistance to an antibiotic, which is why most doctors recommend stopping the medication once the symptoms are gone.

Acne treatment mistakes

For many acne sufferers, the wide variety of treatments and medications can be confusing. With wrong information, it is easy to commit mistakes and aggravate acne condition. Here are some common acne treatment mistakes to avoid.

Not trying acne treatment long enough

Skin may react to products slowly. Acne requires time to heal and improve. Give products at least one month to work and continue to use it if there is any improvement. It is also common to feel a little irritated during the first few days of a treatment. This only means that the product is reacting to the skin. However, these irritations should only be mild, discontinue the use of any products that causes severe side effects.

Over cleaning the skin

Aggravated scrubbing can only worsen acne because it removes the protective skin barrier and can lead to irritation. Use a pH balanced cleanser to clean the face gently. Washing the face more than twice can also strip the skin of its natural oil, making it drier and more susceptible to bacteria.

Trying too many products at once

Trying too many products at once can irritate the skin, especially in products with strong chemicals. Keep your skin regimen clean and simple. Some products also counter act the effects of other treatments. Be sure to consult a dermatologist if you have any serious side effects or want to know more about how a product will affect your skin.

Choosing the wrong products

Harsh cleansers and alcohol based products can worsen acne. People should choose products that do not clog the pores to prevent acne buildup.

Popping and picking acne

Picking on blemishes only prolong its healing process and increases the risk of scarring. Fingers can transfer bacteria to the wound and infect it. This only leads to more swelling. Wait for the pimple to dry out.

Waiting too long to see a dermatologist

Contact a specialist if acne is starting to get out of hand and when treatments do not respond to the acne anymore. Clinics are more equipped to deal with persistent acne and can prescribe stronger medication.

Over-using or under-using medication

Only use medication as instructed. People tend to over use the product in hopes of speeding up its effects, but this will typically just lead to dryness and redness. Some people tend to under use their products because they lose motivation after a few weeks without result. One secret to treating acne is consistency and patience.

Stopping the use of acne products once it clears up

Once acne has subsided, use acne medication less and less rather than abruptly stopping its usage. To keep skin clear and blemish free, people usually have to continue to use one acne product that has been shown to work well for them.

Chapter 2: Acne Removal

Serious acne problems might need certain surgical procedures. People should go through acne removal as a last resort to eliminate acne and the marks that it has left behind. These procedures are mostly done in a doctor's office and should be done under close supervision.

Soft tissue fillers

Collagen is injected into the skin to fill out and flatten any scars while stretching the skin. The effect of these injections is only temporary, so the procedure must be repeated periodically.

Chemical peels

Peels are strong chemicals that are applied on skin to remove the top layer and to even out the skin tone. Peels are effective against shallow acne scars. It is administered by a physician with a cotton ball who spreads the solution on the areas to be targeted. The stronger the consistency of the chemical peel, the deeper it penetrates to the skin and the longer it takes to heal.

Types of chemical peels

Trichloracetic acid(TCA)

This is the mildest chemical peel. TCA is used to reduce the appearance of fine lines and mild blemishes. The pretreatment of Retin A can help TCA penetrate the skin better.

Alphahydroxy Acids(AHA)

AHA is typically a term for a vast array of fruit acid peels like lactic acid, citric, tartaric, malic and glycolic peel. This peel is suited for sun damaged skin and helps eliminate pimples and wrinkles.

Glycolic acid is from sugar cane and is used for mild exfoliation and can help promote collagen production. Citric acid is effective against minor skin damage. Lactic acid peel promotes softer and more radiant skin. Tartaric acid has similar effects to citric acid while malic acid peel is used to treat acne by cleaning the pores.

Phenol

Phenol is a strong chemical peel that is used to treat deep wrinkles and skin discoloration. Phenol can only be used in the face since it can cause scarring on other parts of the body. Also, phenol can only be used for fair skinned individuals because this peel can produce unwanted scarring on darker skin tones.

What to expect from chemical peels

Chemical peel procedure can be as quick as a few minutes. Deep chemical peels may require local anesthesia. The application of the chemical can produce a slight stinging sensation. The skin will be red and can peel afterwards. A cream is usually applied to help heal the skin. It is important to follow the specialist's recommendation to avoid damaging the skin. Chemical peels can be done every few weeks, and treatment is usually based on the condition of the skin.

Dermabrasion

Dermabrasion removes the top layer of the skin with a rotating brush, thereby making space for new layer of skin to grow.

Dermabrasion is not recommended for everyone. People with keloid scars and thin skin should not undergo dermabrasion. Moreover, patients with a viral disease such as oral herpes, are advised to skip dermabrasion since infection can spread during the process and cause permanent scarring.

What to expect from dermabrasion

The procedure can last from 15 minutes to 2 hours. The surgeon will carefully abrade the skin to the agreed depth. An antibiotic ointment will be spread on the face after the procedure to help protect the new skin surface.

The skin is very sensitive after dermabrasion, so it is not advisable to put anything on it without the consent of a dermatologist. It is also highly recommended to avoid sun exposure after a treatment.

Microdermabrasion

This procedure involves a hand-held device that blows crystals into the skin and gently exfoliates the top layer. There is a vacuum that removes the crystals and dead skin cells. The results of this procedure are subtle, but it does decrease the appearance of scars and lessens pimples.

Dermabrasion is effective against scars but not on active acne, so patients have to let their pimples dry first before going through microdermabrasion.

What to expect from microdermabrasion

Microdermabrasion can cause minimal discomfort is rarely painful. The procedure can last up to 40 minutes. Generally, people will need eight treatments to see the desired results. Treatments are usually done in two weeks interval.

Avoid sun exposure and always apply sun screen after treatments. Patients are also advised against exfoliating for a few days after the treatment.

Laser Treatment

Laser treatments can reach deeper into the skin without harming the surface of the skin. It damages the oil glands causing them to produce less oil. Each laser has different wavelengths and color. Facial resurfacing is done with ablative laser that is effective against wrinkles and sun spots. A Non-ablative laser heats up the fibroblast and encourages collagen production instead of removing a layer of the skin.

Types of Laser Treatments

Carbon Dioxide Laser

Carbon dioxide laser treatment is the first ablative laser and is still considered the gold standard for laser treatments. CO_2 lasers can dramatically improve skin texture and tone as well as reduce wrinkles and scars. It involves a recovery period of one month. Hyper pigmentation and redness can occur to darker skin.

Erbium-YAG

This laser penetrates the superficial layers of the skin and dissolves unwanted tissue. The pulsing laser reduces the heat to the skin thereby reducing damage. This is a less invasive option and is effective in improving sun damaged skin. The recovery period is shorter than CO_2 treatments.

Q-switched

Q-switched laser treatments can remove pigmentations and tattoos. It can take eight to twelve sessions to see the desired results.

Fractionated lasers

Fractionated laser treatment is a form of ablative laser that is administered to patients who need stronger treatments. This laser improves the overall skin texture and has the least recovery time of all laser treatments.

What to expect from laser therapy

Laser resurfacing usually takes about 30 minutes to an hour. The exact number of treatments depends on the type of laser being used and the area being treated.

After the laser treatment, an ointment may be applied to the skin to aid the healing process. There will be redness and puffiness in the skin for a few days after the procedure. Keeping the skin moisturized and avoiding sun exposure is important after laser treatment.

Intense Pulsed Light Therapy

Light therapy is said to kill acne causing bacteria. Light treatments also reduce acne scars and can improve the skin texture. IPL uses a broad spectrum light to treat skin conditions like age spots, broken capillaries, tattoos, varicous vein and large pores. There is also less downtime for light therapy.

What to expect from light therapy

The specialist will typically apply topical anesthetic to the affected area. The treatment can be done every three weeks. There might be mild swelling and redness after each treatment. Although uncommon, bleeding can occur after light therapy. There is also a variety of light treatment options available for purchase at stores and on the internet. Blue light has been shown to be the most effective for helping clear up acne.

When to seek acne removal procedures?

People who are overly self-conscious about their acne and acne scars, who also do not respond well to medical or natural remedies, are good candidates for acne removal. Typically, people who have moderate to severe acne find acne removal beneficial and more effective than topical creams. These procedures are great in eliminating blackheads and help diminish large pores.

Benefits

One of the benefits of an acne removal procedure is that a person only has to go through the process a few times in a month. Unlike creams and oral medication that has to be administered continually and religiously, acne removal shows improvement much faster.

Chapter 3: Acne Home Remedies

Acne is a skin problem that affects people of all ages, and although there is no specific cure for acne, there are simple home remedies that can help people get rid of their breakouts.

Fresh grapes

Grapes are rich in antioxidants and polyphenols that can cleanse the skin. It fights pollutants keeping the skin looking young and fresh. Grapes are rich in vitamin C and are effective against inflammation. Rub grape pulp into face to minimize pores.

Cucumber

Cucumber has a cooling and soothing effect that can lessen the inflammation of acne. Cucumber can be directly applied to the affected area or can be mixed with aloe vera and yogurt.

Honey

Honey is a natural antiseptic and has moisturizing properties. Honey can be applied to the face for 30 minutes and it can reduce acne size within a few days. Wash the honey off with warm water when done, and then give your face a quick rinse with cold water to help the pores close. A great brand of honey is: Ambrosia Honey.

Orange peel

Oranges contain acidic properties that can treat acne. The orange juice and the orange peel can both be used to treat acne. The vitamin C in this fruit can also help lighten acne scars.

Indian Lilac

Indian Lilac can be a cure for several different skin problems, including acne. It contains fungicidal properties that can kill bacteria in the skin. Indian lilac is commonly mixed with water and turmeric powder to create a paste before being applied to the face.

Aloe Vera

Aloe Vera juice can treat acne in just a few days. Aloe Vera juice can be applied to the affected area twice a day. It is also effective in reducing acne scars. Most acne products contain aloe vera because of its effective healing properties.

Fenugreek

Fenugreek is an herb that can be used as a treatment for acne. It is an ancient cure for inflammation and contains powerful antioxidants to fight acne causing bacteria. It is usually mixed with water and applied directly to the face.

Tea tree oil

Tea tree oil is an antiseptic that can remove damaged skin cells to make room for new tissue growth. It also has properties that help in treating acne. Apply tea tree oil on the affected area several times a day to minimize it. If you notice redness or irritation then stop usage.

Lemon

Lemon has strong antibacterial properties that can fight pimples. It also has organic acid that can decrease the oil production in the face. Scars and spots can also be reduced by applying lemon juice on the skin.

Natural face masks for acne

Cucumber and Oats Face mask

½ cucumber

2 tbsp oat

Juice of ½ lemon

1 tbsp honey

Cut the cucumber into pieces and put into a blender. Add the oats, lemon juice and honey. Blend the ingredients well until it forms into a paste. Apply to the affected area and leave on for 20 minutes before rinsing off with water.

Apple Cider Vinegar face mask

1 tsp Apple cider vinegar

2 tsp Green tea

1 tsp Honey

5 tsp Sugar

Mix all the ingredients in a small cup. Spread the mask over the face using a cotton pad. Leave it for a few minutes then rinse with warm water.

Cinnamon and Honey face mask

1 tsp cinnamon powder

2 tsp honey

Mix the honey and cinnamon powder until the mixture is thick. Slather it to the face and leave for 15 minutes. Rinse off with warm water.

Turmeric face mask

1 tsp turmeric powder

1 tsp honey

2 tsp milk

Combine all ingredients and mix well. Apply the mixture with a cotton ball to prevent the finger and nails from turning yellow because of the turmeric.

Purifying green tea face mask

3 tbsp green tea

1 tbsp aloe vera gel

1 tbsp honey

2 tbsp kaolin

Green tea face mask helps reduce pores and inflammation. Mix green tea, aloe vera and honey in a bowl. Add the kaolin slowly then stir. Put the mixture in the refrigerator for 10 minutes before applying to the face. This mask can be used once or twice a week.

Lemon face mask

2 tbsp oats

1 tomato

1 tsp lemon juice

Soak the oat in water for a few hours. Squeeze the tomato and add the pulp to the oats. Blend the ingredients together and add the lemon juice. Stir the mixture. Apply on the face and leave for 20 minutes.

Lemon and egg mask

1 egg

5 drops of lemon

Separate the yolk from the egg white. Mix the egg white and lemon juice together. Spread the mixture on the face and leave for 10 minutes. Rinse with cold water then apply moisturizer.

Pumpkin face mask

2 tbsp fresh cream

3 tbsp honey

4 tbsp pumpkin pulp

Mix all ingredients until it has formed a paste. Apply to the face and let it sit for 10 minutes. Apply the face mask once every week for best results.

Baking soda mask

¼ cup water

2 tbsp baking soda

Slowly add water to the baking soda until it forms a paste. Apply to the face using circular motion. Let it dry before rinsing it off with cold water.

Cranberry face mask

¾ cup cranberries

½ cup grapes

4 tsp lemon juice

1 pack gelatin

2 tsp oats

Puree the cranberries and grapes. Mix the gelatin, lemon juice and oats. Mix until it is a thick paste. Put the mixture in the refrigerator for an hour. Apply to the face and let it stay on for 20 minutes. Rinse with water.

Chapter 4: Acne diet

Diet is very important in maintaining an acne free skin. Certain foods can trigger the production of hormones and oil, while others can promote good skin health. Here are some foods that can help clear up acne.

Nettles

Nettles have an anti-inflammatory property that is best taken as a tea. This tea can improve skin complexion and help detoxify the body. It also has high levels of antioxidants that counter acts the effects of free radicals that can damage the tissues and cells of the body.

Peppermint

Peppermint is known for its calming ability. It also aids in digestion and relieves stress. Peppermint tea is also used to treat headaches and clear sinuses. Peppermint is also good for the skin since it helps calm irritation and reduce inflammation.

Beetroot

Beetroot has skin clearing qualities that reduce acne inflammation. The roots are rich in vitamin A, potassium, calcium and magnesium and vitamin E. When combined, these nutrients can speed up the healing process and cleans the toxin out of the body.

Watercress

Watercress leaves are full of antioxidants and minerals that are essential in nourishing the skin and flushing out any impurities. It is rich in potassium, manganese, and carotene.

Tofu

Tofu is a great source for protein; its soft omelet like texture is made from soy beans that are packed with minerals like calcium, iron and healthy fats. These healing properties make a good combination for anyone suffering from acne. It is also an antioxidant that helps cleanse the body.

Dark Berries

Dark berries are a rich source of fiber and antioxidants that can help regulate insulin production. These berries are good for clearing up acne prone skin.

Nuts

Nuts are healthy snacks and the selenium in them helps to increase the production of white blood cells which in turn can help fight bacteria in the body and strengthen the immune system. Nuts are rich in vitamin E, calcium, potassium, and magnesium, which are good for overall skin health.

Brown Rice

Studies have shown that high blood sugar level is linked to acne. Brown rice is a low glycemic alternative to carbohydrate rich food. It also provides protein, magnesium, antioxidants, and vitamin B.

Legumes

Legumes are good for healing acne as they contain potent amounts of vitamins and minerals that can detoxify the body. Legumes are also high in dietary fiber which can help the body's digestion process.

Avocado

Avocado is a rich source of vitamin E which can boost skin health and clarity. It also has vitamin C that can help reduce inflammation. Avocado oil is also believed to stimulate collagen production that improves skin texture and tone.

Tomatoes

Tomatoes are a rich source of vitamin C which can increase collagen production. It also contains lycopene that encourages skin circulation and can help clear out blemishes.

Artichoke

The regular consumption of artichokes is said to improve skin luminosity and prevent acne. It is also a potent herbal remedy because of its antioxidant property. Artichokes also aid digestion and help lower cholesterol, which can help the body's immune system.

Burdock

Burdock has been known throughout the centuries for it healing properties and its high levels of calcium, magnesium and potassium. This herb also has strong antibacterial and antifungal properties that can help stop the spread of acne. Burdock can be eaten or turned into a tea for consumption.

Cottage cheese

Cottage cheese is good for reducing skin acne because it is a rich source of protein and selenium.

Sweet potato

Studies show that high cortisol levels can lead to break-outs. Regulating the blood sugar level can help in balancing out cortisol and thus help reduce stress and break outs. Vitamin packed carbohydrates like sweet potatoes release sugar slowly thereby regulating the blood sugar level. They are also rich in beta carotene which can help the circulation of oxygen into the skin.

Acai

Acai berries are one of the richest sources of antioxidants. They help clear the skin by eliminating toxins and free radicals.

Mackerel

Increase in the consumption of oily fish like the mackerel will promote radiant and spot free skin. It is loaded with eicosapentaenoic and docosahexaeonic acid that can reduce skin inflammation.

Oysters

Oysters are rich in nutrients from vitamin A to zinc. These minerals are essential in maintaining skin health and keeping acne at bay.

Pumpkin seeds

Pumpkin seeds are high in vitamin E and healthy fatty acids, which helps make them effective in fighting acne causing bacteria.

Recipes

Pineapple – Tofu fried rice

- 1 pack tofu, cubed
- 1 tbsp soy sauce
- 2 tbsp cooking sherry
- 2 cloves garlic
- 1 tsp minced ginger
- 2 tbsp olive oil
- 1 cup pineapple juice
- 1 cup peas
- 1 cup diced carrots
- ½ tsp salt
- 3 cups brown rice

- 1 cup pineapple bits

Place tofu in a bowl. Pour the soy sauce and sherry into the tofu and marinate for an hour. Sauté garlic and ginger in olive oil over medium heat. Add in the pineapple juice, carrots, salt and peas. Cook until tender. Add the brown rice, pineapple chunks and tofu and cook for another 5 minutes.

Buckwheat pancakes with bananas

- 1 cup buckwheat flour
- 2 sliced large bananas
- 1 tbsp brown sugar
- ½ tbsp salt
- 2 tbsp potato starch
- 1 tsp baking powder
- 2 tbsp canola oil
- 1 cup rice milk
- Cooking spray
- Brown syrup

Combine all dry ingredients in a bowl. Add the milk and oil then whisk until it is mixed thoroughly. Preheat a pan and spray it with cooking spray. Pour the batter into the pan, evening it out with a spatula. Cook until bubbles appear. Flip and cook on the other side. Serve the pancakes with bananas.

Romaine and Smoked Salmon Salad

1 small organic romaine lettuce

2 diced tomatoes

1 carrot

5 oz thinly sliced smoked salmon

4 sliced radishes

1/2 diced cucumber

Juice of ½ lemon

1 tbsp canola oil

1 tsp ginger root

Place romaine leaves in a plate and top with salmon, carrots, radishes and tomatoes. Mix lemon juice, canola oil and ginger then sprinkle over salad.

Green Pea and Mushroom Risotto

2 tbsp olive oil

4 lb mushrooms

1 diced mushrooms

1 chopped onion

1 2/3 cup brown rice

4 ¼ cup vegetable broth

¼ lb frozen peas

3 tbsp chopped parsley

Salt and pepper to taste

Heat the oil in a large pan. Place the mushrooms in the pan and season with salt and pepper. Stir until mushrooms are tender. Transfer to plate. Heat another 1 tsp of oil and sauté garlic and onion for a few minutes until fragrant. Add the rice and stir constantly. Add a half cup of broth and cook until almost all the liquid is absorbed. Add another half cup of broth towards the end. Add in the peas, mushroom and parsley. Cook for few minutes then season with salt and pepper. Garnish with parsley.

Carrot Fennel Cucumber salad

6 thinly sliced carrots

1 sliced cucumber

1 thinly sliced fennel bulb

1 cup chopped parsley

4 tbsp lemon juice

1 tsp salt

2 tbsp canola oil

1 tsp ground pepper

Mix cucumber, carrots and fennel in a bowl. Combine lemon juice, pepper, salt and oil in a container and stir thoroughly. Pour the dressing over the salad and mix.

Apple and onion soup

1 tbsp chopped rosemary

½ tbsp thyme

1 tbsp canola oil

1 chopped leek

2 sliced onions

3 diced apples

6 cup low sodium vegetable broth

Heat the oil in a pan over medium heat. Sauté the garlic and onions. Add the broth and bring to a boil. Toss in the apples and let it simmer for 10 minutes.

Barley soup with carrots and parsley

2/3 cups water

1/3 cup barley

2 tbsp olive oil

½ cup chopped yellow onion

1 cup carrots

1 2/3 cup plain yogurt

2/3 cup minced parsley

½ tsp black pepper

Salt and pepper to taste

Boil water in a pot then add barley. Cover and simmer for 25 minutes. Remove from heat then set aside. Cook onion in olive oil in a pan until soft. Add the stock and simmer for 20 minutes. Mix in the barley and yogurt. Season then serve.

Sweet potato ginger soup

1 tbsp canola oil

3 large sweet potatoes

2 medium yellow onions

1 chopped ginger

6 cups vegetable broth

Salt and pepper to taste

Heat the oil in a medium pan. Sauté the onions until they are fragrant. Boil the broth then add the sweet potatoes and ginger. Simmer until the potatoes are soft. Puree the soup with a blender until smooth. Season it with salt and pepper. Serve hot.

Chicken and apple salad

3 cups diced cooked chicken

½ cup diced celery

1 cup halved grapes

½ cup diced apples

3 tbsp chopped onion

6 tbsp light mayonnaise

2 tsp lemon juice

Lettuce leaves

Salt and pepper to taste

Combine chicken, grapes, celery, red onion and apples. In a separate bowl mix mayonnaise, lemon juice, salt and pepper, then add to the chicken. Arrange the lettuce leaves and top with the chicken salad.

Salmon Dill Soup

2 medium salmon fillets

2 cups water

1 sweet potato 2 carrots

½ onion

½ cup dill

1 tsp salt

6 tsp cornstarch

Slice salmon into thin strips then set aside. Bring the water to a boil then toss in the sweet potato, onion, and carrots. Cook for 10 minutes. Add the salmon, salt, and dill, and then let it simmer for 3 minutes. In a separate bowl, dissolve the cornstarch into cold water and then pour into the soup. Stir continuously and allow the mixture to thicken. Remove from heat then serve.

Drinks

2 cups chopped fresh pineapples

1 cup green tea

1 tbsp honey

½ chopped fresh ginger

1 cup crushed ice

Combine all ingredients in a blender and process until smooth. Serve cold

Blueberry banana smoothie

1 cup blueberries

1 cup soy milk

1 sliced ripe banana

1 tbsp flaxseed

Mix all ingredients in a food processor. Blend until smooth. Garnish as desired.

Catechin ice tea

2 cups water

2 ½ tsp green tea leaves

3 tbsp organic lemon juice

Bring the water to boil then place the leaves in the pot. Strain the tea and add lemon juice. Refrigerate before serving.

Desserts

Apple slices with cinnamon

1 medium apple

¼ tsp cinnamon

Sprinkle cinnamon on apple and serve immediately.

Carrot Muffins

1 egg

1 cup rice milk

2 cups quinoa flour

1 tsp guar gum

4 tbsp canola oil

1 tbsp flaxseed meal

3 ½ gluten free baking powder

½ tsp salt

¼ cup brown sugar

1 cup grated carrots

¼ cup raisins

1 tsp cinnamon

Preheat the oven. Mix egg, oil and rice milk in a bowl and beat together. Combine the dry ingredients in another bowl.

Slowly pour the liquid ingredients and mix. Fill muffin cups with the batter about two thirds full. Place in the oven and bake for 20 minutes.

Low-fat apple and raspberry crumble

5 large apples

1 cup raspberries

2 cups rolled oats

2 cups apple juice

2 tbsp butter

2 tbsp brown sugar

2 tsp cinnamon

½ tsp cloves

Place apples and blueberries in a baking pan then pour juice over them. Mix oats, sugar and spices in a medium bowl. Cover the apples with toppings and bake for 45 minutes. Serve hot or cold.

Quinoa Crepes with applesauce

1 ½ cup quinoa flour

½ cup tapioca flour

1 tsp cinnamon

1 tsp baking soda

2 cups carbonated water

3 cups apple sauce

3 tbsp canola oil

Cinnamon to taste

Mix quinoa flour, baking soda, cinnamon and tapioca flour in a bowl. Add the water and whisk until smooth. Heat a large pan and pour canola oil. Pour the batter and cook on medium heat. Flip and cook on the other side. Serve with apple sauce.

Fiber Muffins

1 ½ cup bran wheat

1 cup nonfat milk

1 egg

½ cup unsweetened apple sauce

2/3 cup brown sugar

½ cup whole wheat flour

½ cup all purpose flour

1 tsp baking powder

1 tsp baking soda

½ tsp salt

1 cup chopped apples

Combine bran and milk. In a separate bowl, mix apple sauce, bran, and egg. Stir the bran mixture. In a small bowl, mix all purpose flour, baking powder, baking soda, and whole wheat flour. Add the bran mixture and mix. Add the apples. Fill the muffin tins with batter and bake for 20 minutes.

Chapter 5: Acne Control

The skin is the largest organ in the body so it is important to keep it healthy and blemish free as much as possible. Here are some lifestyle changes that can keep acne at bay.

Get more sleep

Stress can increase glucocorticoid production which can cause skin problems like acne. Lack of sleep can aggravate acne and increase inflammation. Sleeping relaxes the body and makes it easier for acne to heal.

Turn the thermostat between 65 to 72 degrees Fahrenheit. Lying in a cooler temperature makes it easier to fall asleep.

Limit sugar

In general, avoid food that causes spikes in the blood sugar level because this can result in inflammation. Excess levels of insulin can trigger a hormonal cascade that can lead to the growth of bacteria and the production of oil. Studies have shown that people who are in a low-glycemic diet have fewer breakouts.

Exercise

Exercise reduces stress, regulates hormones, and increases blood circulation, which helps clear the skin through sweating. Be careful though, sweat can also cause acne. Be sure to wash your face with water after every workout session and wash garments regularly.

Drink water

Water flushes toxins out of the body. Just by drinking two glasses of water, you can increase blood flow throughout the entire body. Flushing out your body with water helps get rid of waste, which makes it easier for the body to fight acne causing bacteria and maintain healthy skin. After trying a variety of different water sources, my all-time favorite is: ZeroWater.

Sunscreen

The sun can do more damage than burning the skin; it can also aggravate pimples and potentially worsen the condition. Acne sufferers should opt for a lighter sunscreen that contains oxybenzone and avobenxone. Avoid products that contain titanium oxide and zinc oxide, since these tend to be thicker in consistency and can block pores. Look for 'noncomedogenic' on the label to make sure that the product does not block the pores.

Consume Omega 3 fatty acids

Good fats like omega 3 fatty acids control the production of leukotriene B4, a molecule that increases the oil production. A good source of Omega 3 is **Nature Made Fish Oil Omega 3**.

Washing your face

Wash your face twice a day to clear the skin of sweat, dirt, and makeup that can lead to acne breakouts. Make it a habit to wash the face in the morning and night with gentle cleanser.

Use the right product for your skin type. Drier skin needs products that do not rob the skin of too much oil while oily skin needs a stronger formula.

Exfoliate and Moisturize

Gently exfoliate the skin once a week to remove dead skin cells that can also be the breeding ground for bacteria. A body loofah is great for this. Follow up with a moisturizer to help protect the skin and to replenish the lost moisture after each wash.

Astringent

If you notice your skin is oily or are in a rush and don't want to wash your face, applying a deep cleaning astringent to your face with a cotton ball or paper towel is excellent for treating acne.

Clean your cellphone

Studies have shown that cellphones are a breeding ground for germs. They can be exposed to thousands of bacteria that can be passed from the fingers to the face. The heat produced by the phone also aids the multiplication of bacteria. Wipe your phone with hand sanitizer every day.

Sleep with a clean face

Remove makeup before sleeping. Makeup can clog the pores that lead to acne. Invest in some wipes that can be used to clean your face without water.

Stop touching your face

Fingers can be a breeding ground for bacteria so avoid touching your face to prevent it from transferring.

Keep it clean

Change pillowcases and towels weekly to prevent bacteria from building up and causing breakouts.

Pay attention to hair routine

The scalp releases oil to keep the hair shiny and lustrous. Too much oil can seep from the hair to the skin. Try to wash your hair every other day to prevent acne. Too much products such as gels and sprays can also get into pores and clog them. Be careful in applying hair products, especially to the forehead. Consider non-fragrant products to clean your hair. Also, make sure to rinse conditioner thoroughly from your hair, as it may contain oil that can transfer to the skin.

Check laundry detergent

Laundry detergents also contain harsh chemicals that can cause breakouts. Opt for natural laundry detergents instead.

Reduce stress

Stress is linked to breakouts. Try to maintain a happy and calm disposition to control acne. Do recreational and enjoyable things to look and feel better.

Quit smoking and drinking

Smoking and excessive drinking can dehydrate the skin which makes it prone to acne breakouts. Eliminating these habits can make the body so much healthier. If you need help with this be sure to check out my books: **Quit Smoking Now Quickly and Easily** and my other book **Influence, Willpower, and Discipline**.

Make up tips for concealing acne

Acne cannot be cured overnight so concealing them temporarily is essential in looking fresh and clean.

Step 1

Wash your face with a medicated cleanser. Gently scrub the skin in a circular motion then rinse with cold water. Apply toner then moisturize with a water based moisturizer.

Step 2

Choose a tinted moisturizer to conceal mild acne. Tinted moisturizer can help reduce the appearance of acne. Use your fingers to dab a small amount onto the face and then blend it in a circular motion. Do not try to cover all blemishes; just create a base layer that can cover mild imperfections.

Step 3

Use a concealer brush to apply liquid concealer. Apply a very small amount directly on the blemish. Choose a shade that is slightly lighter than the skin tone. Use a green primer to counteract the redness of acne.

You can conceal oily acne with powder. Use a powder brush to apply powder and set the makeup. Both translucent and tinted powder works well in covering blemishes.

Conclusion

I hope this book was able to help you to understand how to cure and prevent acne. Acne can be a real nuisance and sometimes it can take weeks or even months to get the desired results. Don't give up! Find out which strategies work best for you and then use them several times per day. Keep a journal of foods you eat, so you can tell which foods may be giving you break outs. With patience and persistence you can defeat your acne problems once and for all!

Finally, if you discovered at least one thing that has helped you or that you think would be beneficial to someone else, be sure to take a few seconds to easily post a quick positive review. As an author, your positive feedback is desperately needed. Your highly valuable five star reviews are like a river of golden joy flowing through a sunny forest of mighty trees and beautiful flowers! *To do your good deed in making the world a better place by helping others with your valuable insight, just leave a nice review.*

Thanks and Best of Luck

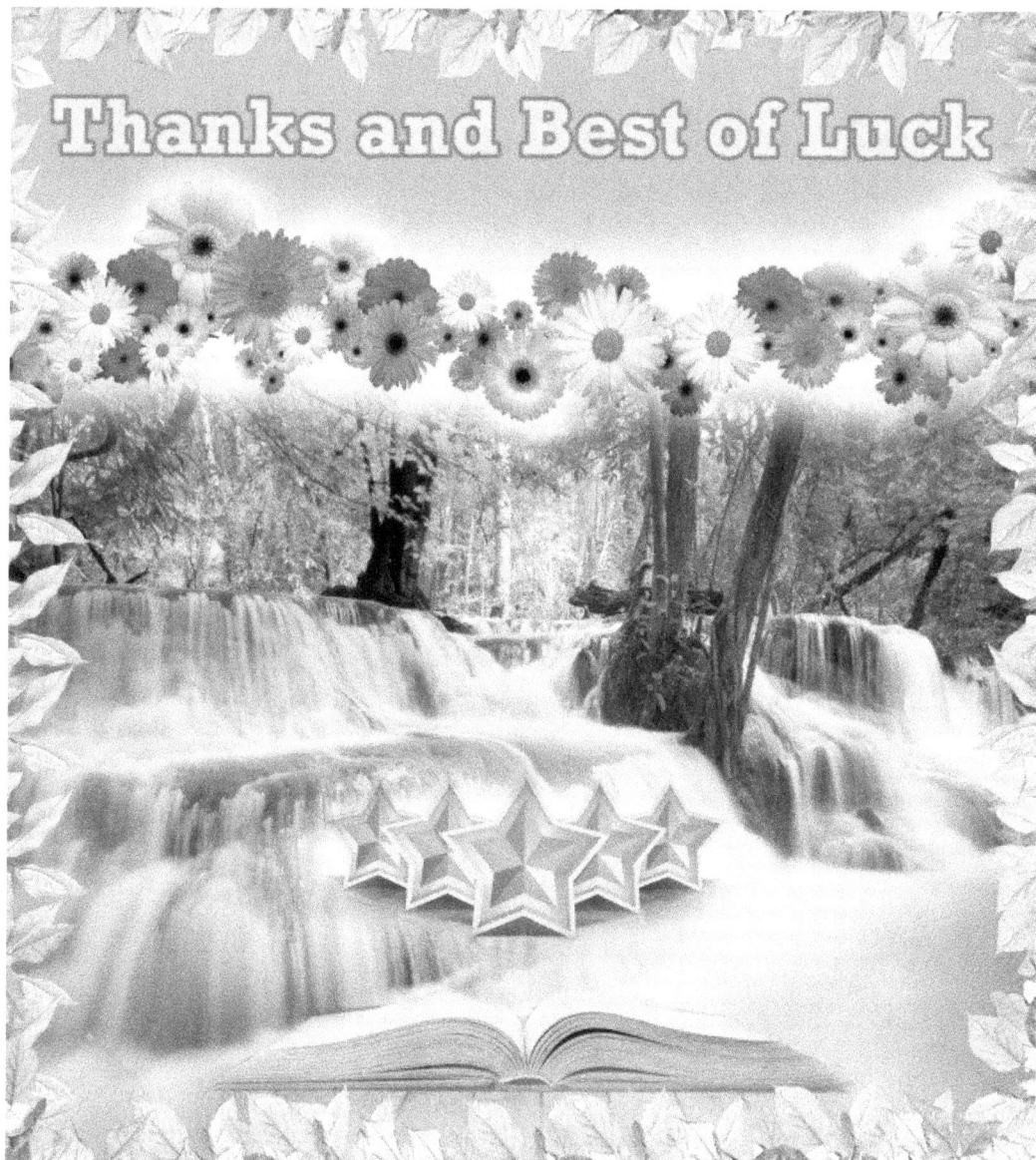

My Other Books and Audio Books
www.AcesEbooks.com

Health Books

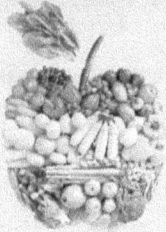

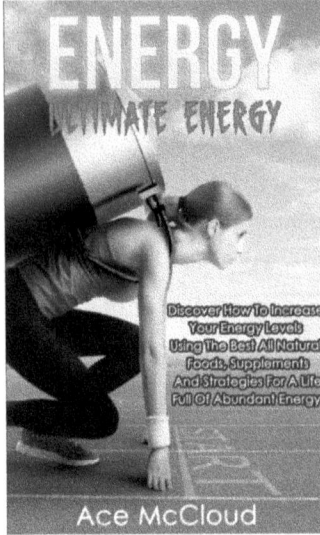

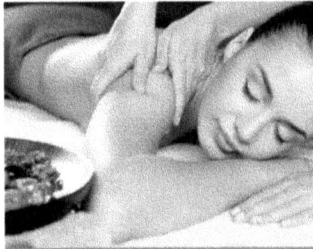

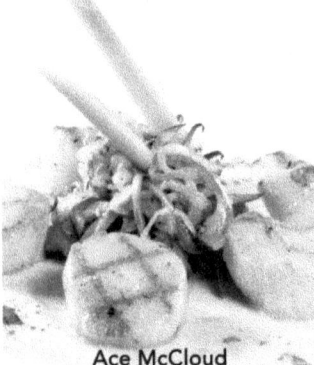

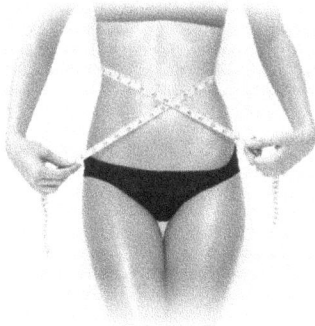

LOSE WEIGHT

THE TOP 100 BEST WAYS
TO LOSE WEIGHT QUICKLY AND HEALTHILY

Ace McCloud

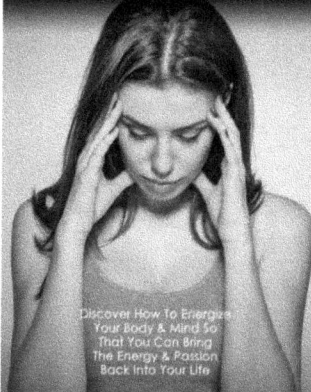

FATIGUE

OVERCOME CHRONIC FATIGUE

Discover How To Energize
Your Body & Mind So
That You Can Bring
The Energy & Passion
Back Into Your Life

Ace McCloud

Peak Performance Books

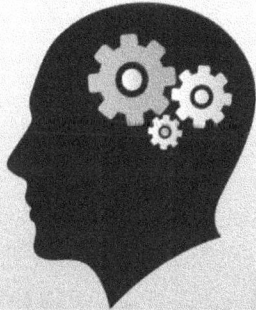

SUCCESS

SUCCESS STRATEGIES

THE TOP 100 BEST WAYS TO BE SUCCESSFUL

Ace McCloud

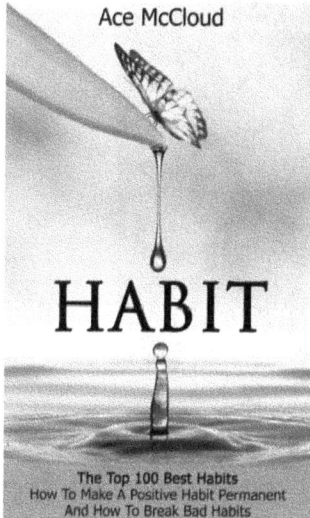

Ace McCloud

HABIT

The Top 100 Best Habits
How To Make A Positive Habit Permanent
And How To Break Bad Habits

MOTIVATION

MASTER THE POWER OF MOTIVATION
TO PROPEL YOURSELF TO SUCCESS

Ace McCloud

ATTITUDE

Discover The True Power Of
A Positive Attitude

Ace McCloud

SELF DISCIPLINE

Unleash The Power Of Self Discipline,
Influence And Willpower In Your Life
To Achieve Anything

Ace McCloud

Competitive Strategies

WINNING STRATEGIES

The Top 100 Best Strategies
For Peak Performance During Competitions

Ace McCloud

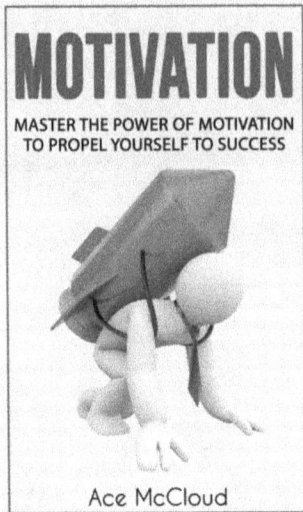

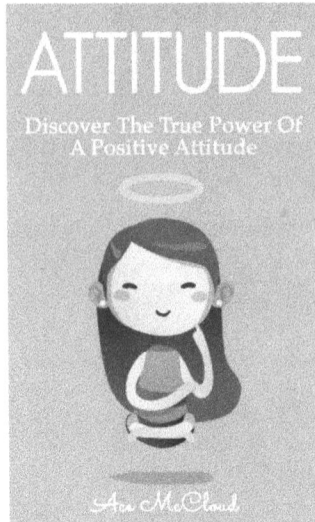

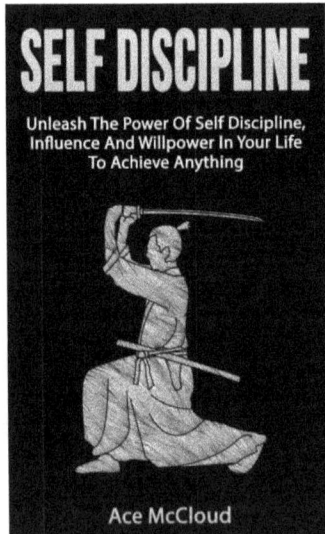

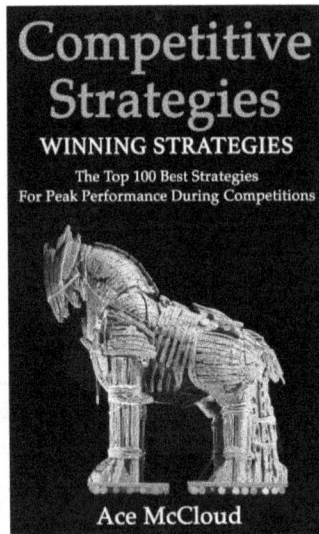

Be sure to check out my audio books as well!

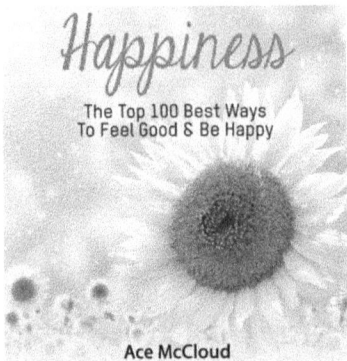

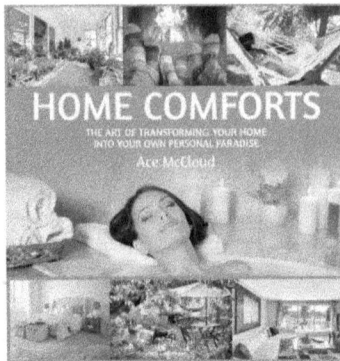

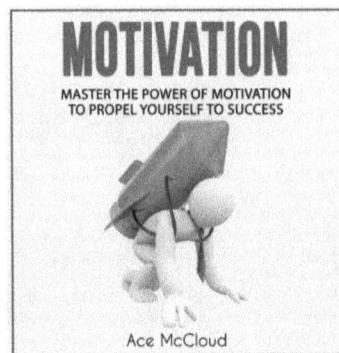

Happiness

The Top 100 Best Ways
To Feel Good & Be Happy

Ace McCloud

HOME COMFORTS

THE ART OF TRANSFORMING YOUR HOME
INTO YOUR OWN PERSONAL PARADISE

Ace McCloud

MOTIVATION

MASTER THE POWER OF MOTIVATION
TO PROPEL YOURSELF TO SUCCESS

Ace McCloud

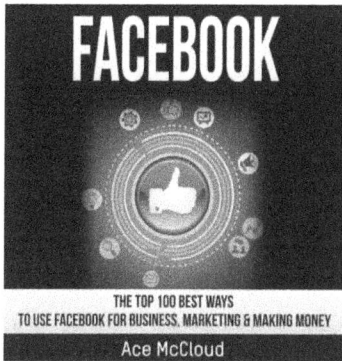

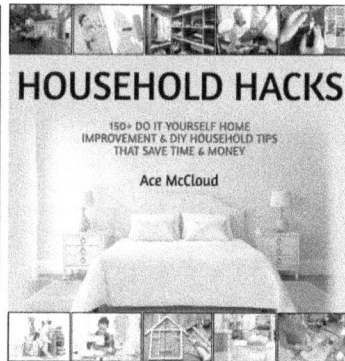

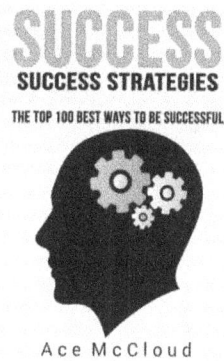

Be sure to check out my website at: www.AcesEbooks.com for a complete list of all of my books and high quality audio books. I enjoy bringing you the best knowledge in the world and wish you the best in using this information to make your journey through life better and more enjoyable! **Best of luck to you!**

www.ingramcontent.com/pod-product-compliance
Lightning Source LLC
Chambersburg PA
CBHW080632030426
42336CB00018B/3164